Wilderness
Survival

∕ιFALCONGUIDE®

Wilderness Survival

STAYING ALIVE UNTIL HELP ARRIVES

Second Edition

Suzanne Swedo

FALCONGUIDE®

GUILFORD, CONNECTICUT
HELENA, MONTANA

AN IMPRINT OF THE GLOBE PEQUOT PRESS

For Rex

AFALCONGUIDE ®

Illustrations by Todd Telander

Library of Congress Cataloging-in-Publication Data is
available.
ISBN-13: 978-0-7627-4012-3
ISBN-10: 0-7627-4012-4

Manufactured in the United States of America
Second Edition/First Printing

Contents

Acknowledgments

Special thanks to Ron Hood for reviewing the manuscript and for striking the spark, to Brad Childs at the Wilderness Institute, Melinda Goodwater and Singaman Lama of Goodwater's Adventures, Jim Lowery of Earth Skills, and Steve Tabor of Desert Survivors. I appreciate help from the National Outings Program of the Sierra Club and Marie Cecchini of its Rocky Mountains subcommittee, Carol Dienger of its Alaska subcommittee, and Lettie French, Andy Johnson, and Jim Watters with the Knapsack subcommittee. Also, thanks to the organizers of the Angeles Chapter of the Basic Mountaineering Training and Wilderness Training Course. Thanks to Penny Otwell and Steve Medley at the Yosemite Association. For assistance in the field, special thanks to John Alderson, Betty Berenson, Craig Deutsche, Laura Lathrop, and Rex Raymer.

Introduction

Most backcountry travelers set out into the wilderness for recreation, love of nature, or self-discovery and to experience the sense of freedom that comes from breaking out of the technological and social cocoon that feeds and shelters them—and separates them from the natural world. That freedom has a price, however. Wilderness, by definition, is a place without easy access to the facilities and services established to keep people out of trouble or rescue them when they get into it. In the wilderness you are on your own and expected to be both mentally and materially self-sufficient.

Most wilderness areas in North America are under the jurisdiction of some public agency—such as the USDA Forest Service, the National Park Service, Parks Canada, or the Bureau of Land Management—that is equipped to help people in emergencies. These agencies recognize that accidents can happen to even the most skilled and experienced outdoorspeople. Still, such agencies are usually understaffed and underfunded and already busy enough protecting the wilderness from destruction by visitors rather than the other way around. Many national parks, for example, which formerly conducted helicopter rescues for free, are now forced to charge victims for the service, and a very expensive service it is.

Increasingly, the use of cell phones to summon aid for people who have gotten into trouble through their own carelessness, ignorance, or lack of preparation has strained to the limit the resources of search-and-rescue organizations, many of which are staffed by volunteers. That is not to say that cell phones have no place in the backcountry, but they should not be used as substitutes for personal responsibility.

Using This Book

This book is intended to help you survive short-term wilderness emergencies, to help you learn what to do when you become lost or stranded by bad weather, or you are forced to jettison your pack when you fall in a river, or you survive a plane crash in some remote area. Such emergencies are almost always resolved within a very few days, so you don't need to learn to tan hides or chip spear points, though such skills may be very satisfying to master. What you will learn here is how to safely and comfortably enjoy the backcountry, how to avoid common wilderness mishaps, and how to handle them when they arise.

Before you go, read this book to get an idea of the wilderness situations that can arise, then carry the book with you for reference. Remember, though, that reading a book is not enough in itself. Practice your wilderness skills and techniques at home first. Then get all the experience you can with knowledgeable people. Many community colleges, city and county recreation departments, and wilderness organizations such as the Sierra Club, Mountaineers, Appalachian Mountain Club, schools such as NOLS (National Outdoor Leadership School), Outward Bound, and other private organizations offer wilderness-skills programs.

Before You Go

PORTRAIT OF A SURVIVOR

The most important characteristic shared by survivors of wilderness emergencies is a positive attitude. Almost invariably, people who come through harrowing experiences unscathed are those who believe they will. They are the people who see an emergency as a problem to solve, a challenge to overcome, who never even consider the possibility of failure.

People survived and flourished for about two million years before modern civilization, and each of us still possesses that most effective and versatile of survival tools—a human brain. If you can overcome the mindless panic that sometimes rears up in scary situations and gets in the way of your common sense, your chances of finding a way out of danger increase enormously.

In addition to the possession of a "can do" attitude, those most likely to overcome dangers to life and limb are people with a strong sense of *personal responsibility*. The wilderness is neither benevolent nor hostile; it really doesn't care one way or the other about you. It is up to you to take care of yourself, plan carefully, equip yourself properly, be physically fit, know basic first aid, and accept the consequences of your actions. Do not set off into the wilderness alone. Two people are the minimum, but the ideal number for a traveling group is four. In case of illness or injury,

---

When faced with some potential disaster, stop, calm down, and think.

---

one person can remain with the victim while the other two go for help. If you are inexperienced, first seek experienced companions, join a group, take a class, and do some reading.

Assess your physical condition honestly. Do you do any kind of vigorous, regular (at least three times weekly) aerobic activity? Nature favors the strong. You don't need to be an athlete, but you should be fit and healthy. Walking on level ground in city or suburbs bears almost no resemblance to negotiating rocky, sandy, muddy, steeply ascending or descending wild country. Try a few full-day hikes over varied terrain, then a weekend outing or two before tackling a week-long expedition.

Investigate carefully the full range of conditions you might encounter in an area during the time of year you plan to visit, and choose equipment accordingly. Remember that the finest and most expensive gear in the world can't insure you against errors in judgment or lack of knowledge. On the other hand, do not practice false economy on items that ensure your safety and comfort, such as tents and sleeping bags. If you cannot afford to buy good equipment, you probably can rent it in your hometown or in cities and towns near popular wilderness areas. Consult wilderness veterans about gear, study magazines and catalogs, and shop at reputable wilderness outfitters whose salespeople use the equipment themselves.

Test equipment at home first: Fire up your stove; pitch your tent in the backyard. Don't get caught in the dark in a howling storm trying to make sense of yards of flapping nylon, miles of tangled tent cord, and an impossible number of poles poking out in a dozen different directions.

Pretrip Checklist

• *Leave word, preferably in writing, with someone at home about your planned itinerary and time of return.*

• *Check weather forecasts for the area you plan to visit.* High mountains create their own local weather, and conditions that could affect you might not show up on the national satellite weather map on television or in the newspaper. Be careful not to get caught at high altitude in a bad storm or along a stream in a flash flood. For more information see the FalconGuide *Reading Weather* by Jim Woodmencey.

• *Find out whom to contact at the nearest trailhead in case of emergency.* In national parks it will be the National Park Service, but in other areas the sheriff's office is your best bet. Make a mental note of the location of the phone nearest the trailhead.

• *Check for current conditions or possible hazards on your route with local authorities, usually the district ranger.* Is there recent rockslide or avalanche damage, washed-out bridges or high water, bear activity? Be aware.

• *Double-check your equipment checklist to make sure you packed everything, including the Ten Essentials (see page 10).*

• *Make sure you have a permit if the local managing agency requires one.*

WILDERNESS PERMITS

Most national parks and national forests require visitors to pick up a wilderness permit before entering a wilderness area. This is your opportunity to find out everything you need to know. Wilderness permits are sometimes free; sometimes a nominal fee is charged. You must state the day and place you plan to enter and leave the wilderness and provide an estimated itinerary. Your signature on this permit does not mean you have hired local rangers as babysitters. Nobody will come looking for you if you do not return on time unless you have left word with someone at home to do so. If you do not show up as expected, friends or relatives can contact the ranger station to begin a search based on the information on your permit.

The Ten or More Essentials

The list of Ten Essentials was originally compiled by the Mountaineers of Seattle, and its use is recommended by other wilderness hiking and mountaineering organizations, including the Sierra Club. It should be considered a guide only; if your travels take you into wilderness areas other than the mountains of the West, such as tropical or desert regions, you probably should add or delete various items.

These essentials should accompany you on a wilderness outing of any length, from a day hike lasting a few hours to an extended expedition. They should be attached to your body in some way, perhaps in a pouch attached to your belt. They shouldn't be packed away in your backpack because their purpose is to keep you safe and relatively comfortable in the absence of any other gear.

THE TEN ESSENTIALS

1. Extra Food and Water

Extra food means food that is not part of a planned meal or snack, food you do not expect to eat. So you won't be tempted to eat it except in case of emergency, it probably should not be one of your favorites. It does not have to be a large quantity. It probably will not keep you from starving, but it might give you some comfort as well as a few calories to burn to keep you warm. One or two high-energy sports bars might be a good choice.

Always carry a full liter of water, and keep it full. Refill at every water source. The next source may be a long way off.

2. Extra Clothing

This, too, is gear you do not expect to use. A polypropylene or wool sweater is fine. Even better is a small Mylar space blanket, the kind that comes folded up in a little cellophane package about 2 inches by 4 inches. Add a couple of thirty-gallon trash bags, 2 or 3 millimeters thick if you can find them. These are extremely compact, weigh practically nothing, and can be tucked into your emergency kit and forgotten until needed. Garbage bags make good rain and wind protection. They can also be used for gathering food, for insulation, as fire-making material, for forming part of a shelter, or for melting snow.

3. Map

A topographic map is essential for wilderness navigation. It also can be tucked inside your clothes for insulation or used to leave notes or directions addressed to potential rescuers.

4. Compass

Be sure you know how to use both a map and compass or they won't do you much good. If your compass is the type with a mirror, it can double as a signaling device.

5. Flashlight with Extra Batteries and Bulb

A small AA-battery light is fine. Its most important use is for reading a map and perhaps for signaling. A headlamp that keeps your hands free is the most convenient and usually the smallest and lightest in weight. The LED type is brighter and conserves batteries longer than the kind with a standard bulb. You will probably find that if it is absolutely necessary to walk after dark, starlight alone provides enough light once your night vision adjusts and you are sure of your footing.

6. Sunglasses and Sunscreen

These might not be critical for wandering through the Eastern woods, but they are absolutely essential for survival in deserts, on snow, or in high mountains above timberline where the atmosphere is thin. Sunburn can lead to severe dehydration. The same conditions can cause snow blindness, a particularly painful, though usually temporary, condition that can occur within less than an hour's exposure, though the symptoms may not show up until eight hours later.

7. Matches in a Waterproof Container

The wooden strike-anywhere variety is best. Just be sure to store them in such a way that they cannot rub against one another and light themselves. An airtight pill bottle or film canister will keep both oxygen and water out.

8. Fire Starter or Candle

In rain or wind a match will not stay lit long enough to ignite damp tinder. A candle, even a small piece of candle at least a half-inch in diameter, will give a more lasting flame. Better yet is fire starter, available at outfitting stores in several forms, from tablets or small blocks of paraffin or other flammable material to a gel that squeezes from a tube.

9. Pocket Knife or Utility Tool

One simple blade will do, though the models with scissors, saws, tweezers, screwdrivers, and other utility tools are handy for preparing tinder, preparing food, first aid, equipment repair, and almost any other task you can imagine.

10. First-Aid Kit

Your kit should include a few alcohol swabs or moist towelettes, antibiotic ointment, aspirin or ibuprofen, Band-Aids, small tweezers, and scissors. Also include whatever prescription drugs you take regularly. If you travel alone or carry the main kit for a group, take a more elaborate kit. See the FalconGuide *Wilderness First Aid* by Gilbert Preston for a thorough discussion of wilderness first-aid kits.

Some Other Essentials

• Water Purification Device or Chemical

When the Ten Essentials list was originally assembled, water from free-flowing streams was safe to drink in most wilderness areas. That's not always true anymore. Keep some iodine in your emergency kit (as long as you are not allergic to it) whether or not you travel with a filter in your pack.

• Duct Tape

This versatile item can be used for everything from blister protection to equipment repair. At home or in the wilderness, it's easily stored by wrapping a yard or two around a water bottle, match container, pencil, or flashlight.

- **Whistle**

Much more audible than a human voice when signaling for help, a whistle also doesn't wear out as quickly.

- **20-gauge Wire**

Another versatile item, wire can be used for everything from repairs to rigging a tarp. Several feet can be wound into a compact coil that weighs almost nothing and takes up little space.

- **Extra Eyeglasses**

If you are absolutely dependent on eyeglasses, carry a small repair kit (sold in many stores) that contains a tiny screwdriver, screws, and a magnifying glass. Make sure the screws fit your glasses. It is also a good idea just to bring an extra pair of glasses.

A Nonessential

- **Cell Phone**

They don't work in remote areas or even in not-so-remote areas if you're surrounded by rock. They also rely on batteries that may fail. Satellite phones work almost everywhere but are expensive, heavy, and also depend on batteries. There are no substitutes for care and competence.

How Not to Get Lost

Search-and-rescue teams are summoned to find lost people more frequently than for any other reason. The first law of wilderness travel is to pay attention. Take frequent note of significant landmarks and your position in relation to them. Pick features that are visible from a distance, that are big enough and distinctive enough to recognize from all directions. A split tree with a big rock beside it will look like thousands of others when you're unsure of where you are, especially if you're approaching it from a different angle. Which way is the river flowing? Have you been following it upstream or down? Are you on the cooler, damper (usually the northern) side of a slope or on the warmer, drier (usually southern) side? Glance back over your shoulder every now and then to make mental snapshots of the way you came. Should you become confused and have to turn around, at least something will look familiar.

Anticipate the route ahead as well. A common phenomenon in the mountains is a perfectly distinct path through forested country that vanishes altogether at the edge of a meadow. Stop and scan the far side. Are there gaps in the trees beyond? Where would the most likely spot be for the trail to continue? Once you've wandered absentmindedly into the center of a field, you're likely to lose track of the way you came as well as the way you intended to go. Keep an eye out for markers such as downed trees or logs in which a gap has been sawed, especially if there is a series of them.

TRAIL MARKERS

Watch for man-made trail markers. Cairns, also known as ducks, are piles of rocks that indicate a trail. They may be used to show a route over bare rock slabs or to mark where a path begins again on the far side of a meadow. There may be no more than two or three fist-size stones on top of one another, so you need to be alert, though in the Arctic or on high mountains where clouds make for poor visibility, a cairn may be as tall as a person.

Blazes are marks made on trees by cutting away the outer bark, usually in simple geometric shapes at approximately eye level. They indicate a trail's location when snow or plant debris covers the forest floor. The scar usually remains for the life of the tree, but occasionally the surrounding bark begins to obscure its outline. If you're uncertain whether you're seeing a blaze or a natural mark, check the opposite side of the tree. Trees are almost always blazed on both sides so they will be visible from either direction. While blazing doesn't usually injure a tree fatally, it does invite disease and infection, so recently constructed trails are more likely to be marked with small metal plates, usually diamond-shaped, instead of blazes.

KEEPING TRACK OF TIME

Another habit worth cultivating for safety is staying aware of the passage of time. There is no shame in wearing a watch in the outdoors any more than there is in using a map and compass. It may be important to your safety to know how many hours of light remain so you can judge whether to cross the next ridge, stop and prepare a warm bivouac for the night, or return to your starting point.

If, however, you have lost, broken, or left your watch at home, you can still get a rough estimate of when the sun will set by extending one arm out in front of you, full length, and bending your wrist so your palm is at a right angle to your arm, facing you. Keeping your fingers stiff and straight and together, move your hand until the edge appears to rest on the horizon. Each finger, on average, covers about 15 minutes of time; each full hand, not counting your thumb,

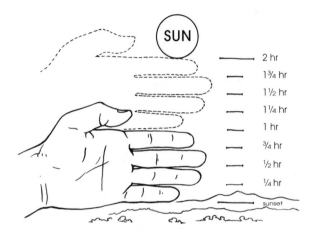

Estimating time until sunset

covers one hour. The number of hand widths between the sun's current position and the horizon is the number of hours remaining until sunset.

It's always good survival practice to note the time whenever you set out on a journey. Learn how long it takes you to cover a mile over different kinds of terrain. The average hiker walks 2.5 to 3 miles per hour on trail over relatively level ground; the average backpacker covers about 2 miles per hour. For every 1,000 feet you gain in elevation, you'll move about 1 mile per hour slower. Cross-country (off-trail) travel is considerably more time-consuming, since it requires constantly picking your way around or over obstacles or pausing to check map and compass bearings.

TOPOGRAPHIC MAPS

The maps most useful to wilderness travelers are the 7.5-minute topographic maps published by the United States Geological Survey (USGS) and the Canada Map Office. These are available at local outfitters or by contacting:

USGS Information Services
P.O. Box 25286
Federal Center
Denver, CO 80225
(303) 202–4700
www.store@usgs.gov

Canada Map Office
130 Bentley Road
Ottawa, Ontario K1A 0E9
Canada
(800) 465–6277

The USGS maps' 7.5-minute format corresponds to the way scientists divide the earth into segments for reference. The earth is divided into two sets of 360 degrees; one set of degrees runs north to south, from pole to pole; the other runs east to west all around the earth's circumference. Each degree is further divided into 60 minutes, each minute into 60 seconds. Thus, these USGS maps cover 7.5 square minutes of the surface of the earth.

The usual scale of USGS maps is 1:24,000; that is, 1 inch on the map equals 24,000 inches, or 2,000 feet, on the ground. Each map covers between 50 and 70 square miles.

The maps are color coded. Green is for vegetation, blue for water-related features, black for human-created structures such as roads and buildings, and brown for topographic features. Updated maps show changes in purple. You can see at a glance where water flows all year and where it flows only in the rainy season, where there are snowfields, glaciers, marshes, or swamps. Patterns of green represent forests, scrub, orchards, and vineyards. Upon request, the USGS will send you a sheet of topographic map symbols with a key that shows what each symbol means.

How Are Topographic Maps Different?

The brown contour lines distinguish "topo" maps from other types. When these contour lines are read properly, they provide very specific information about terrain.

At the bottom of most topo maps, below the scale, is the phrase "Contour Interval 40 Feet" (or 20 feet, or 50 feet). This tells you that the space between each of the brown lines represents 40 feet in elevation. Each line designates terrain that is 40 feet higher or lower than terrain designated by its neighboring line. Every fifth line is a little darker than the others, and the elevation is printed somewhere along it. Contour lines show you at a glance the size and shape of every bump and gully on the land (as long as it's bigger than 40 feet). If the lines are widely spaced, the terrain slopes only gradually; if they're crowded closely together, the land is steeper.

To determine whether you are going uphill or downhill, look for the elevation figures on the darker index lines. Also, since the contour lines form V shapes whenever a stream crosses them, the apex of the V always points upstream.

With practice, you can translate topographic map symbols into a rich and detailed view of the terrain. Develop the habit of carrying your map with you—in your hand, not your pocket—and stop to glance frequently from map to terrain and back again. Once the translation becomes automatic, you'll always know where you are.

COMPASS

A compass enables you to find your way when weather or deep forest prevents navigating by visible landmarks, when there are no landmarks, or when you haven't been paying attention. You can use compass bearings to communicate directions to another person—or to settle arguments about which distant mountain peak is which.

The best kind of compass to learn to use is the orienteering type, but even the simplest is adequate. All you need is one that is mounted on a rectangular baseplate with a moveable ring marked off in increments of usually two to five degrees. Inside the ring, the centered magnetic arrow always points north. (Well, nearly north. More about that later.) On the baseplate outside the ring is an arrow called the "direction-of-travel arrow." On more elaborate compasses there may be some kind of sighting device instead of a simple arrow, but the purpose is the same.

To take a bearing, that is, to find the degrees of direction from where you are to where you're going, aim the direction-of-travel arrow at some feature of the landscape, hold the compass steady and level with one hand, and with the other, rotate the dial so that the 0-degree (or 360-degree) mark is lined up exactly with the floating north-pointing arrow. Then read the number on the dial that matches up with the direction-of-travel arrow. That's your bearing. You can draw that bearing on your map, using your compass as a protractor, to indicate, for example, where on the road you left your car when you went off to climb a peak or in which direction to set out when your final destination is hidden behind a ridge. You also can find out where you are by taking two or three bearings on known features on the land and drawing lines between them on your map. You'll be wherever the lines intersect. There are almost limitless applications that will become obvious to you as soon as you have learned even a little about navigating.

WHEN NORTH ISN'T NORTH

The north on your map isn't the same north as the one on your compass. Maps, by convention, are printed with true north at the top where all the lines of longitude converge at the poles. Compasses, on the other hand, are magnets. Their arrows point to the magnetic North Pole, not the "true" North Pole. The difference between magnetic north and true north is called declination and differs from place to place. For example, in Los Angeles the declination is 14 degrees, while in Fairbanks, Alaska, it is nearer 30 degrees. You have to make an adjustment for declination every time you use your map and compass together.

There are all kinds of mathematical formulas you can use to add or subtract the proper number of degrees from every bearing you take, but there is a much simpler method. In the lower left-hand corner of USGS topographic maps is a drawing of an angle consisting of a side that points to geographic or true north and a side labeled "MN" that points to magnetic north.

The number of degrees in the angle is printed between sides. If you have the kind of compass that allows adjustments, you can adjust it to read 15 degrees (if the true north line is west of you) or 345 degrees (if true north is east of you), for instance, instead of 0 degrees so the readings will agree with your map.

Using another method, you can line up a straight-edge along the magnetic north side of the angle printed on the bottom of the map and continue that line all the way to the top of the map with a pencil. Just use that line instead of the margins of the map (which represent true north and south) as your reference point. Your map and compass will agree, and you can forget about declination.

Modern locator devices such as Global Positioning Systems (GPS) give coordinates of precisely where you are on your map. Knowing those coordinates is useless, though, unless you have a map and know how to read it. If you are injured or stranded, GPS coordinates won't help you if you can't communicate with rescuers. They use a lot of batteries, too.

Even if this all sounds complicated, remember that it is only intended to give you an idea of the possibilities. You won't become proficient at navigation in a few minutes (or even a few hours) or by reading a couple of pages. Take a class, read one of the excellent books available on the subject, and practice, practice, practice.

If You Get Lost

It can happen to anybody. Your light plane goes down in unknown country, or your map blows away and you step on your compass, or, more likely, you've been strolling along in a reverie and suddenly realize that nothing looks familiar. Your map doesn't seem to make any sense, and there is nothing in sight on which to take a compass bearing.

Before you do anything at all, stop. Calm down. Take a few deep breaths.

Trace your way backward in your mind. You've probably noticed more than you realize and can figure out where you went wrong, as long as you haven't allowed panic to interfere with your thinking. There is a common and deadly impulse to run when people find themselves in frightening situations. More than one wilderness tragedy has resulted when someone became disoriented and blindly rushed farther and farther away from camp, trail, or companions.

If you're suddenly overcome by doubts about your position and have been traveling along a trail, a ridge, a stream—or if you can follow your own tracks back the way you came—turn around and retrace your steps until you're sure of your whereabouts, then start out again. Resist the impulse to push ahead while hoping to pick up the trail or to spot some familiar landmark. It's frustrating to waste time going back, but it's quicker than becoming more and more lost.

IF YOU ARE TRULY LOST

If nothing works, if you have decided you are (well and truly) lost, not just temporarily off-route, you have a critical decision to make: to stay or to go. There are a few circumstances in which your best chance is to try to walk out.

When to Walk Out

You should walk out only if one or more of the following are true:

- The area you're in is unsafe.

- Bad weather is approaching and you have no shelter.

- Nobody knows you're missing, so there is no chance of a search being launched.

- You're someplace where a signal is not likely to be noticed.

Find a high point from which to survey the surroundings. Are there any roads, major rivers, or signs of habitation? Sometimes it's useful to follow a major watercourse downstream since people tend to settle and to travel on rivers and along coastlines, but many rivers flow farther and farther into wild country, while others plunge over cliffs too dangerous to negotiate. Acquaint yourself with the courses of major waterways before you set out.

When to Stay Put

In most cases your best bet is to stay where you are and signal for help. Search-and-rescue teams know what to look for, and good trackers can read the signs of your passing in a way that seems positively uncanny. Don't make their job more difficult by changing your location unless it's absolutely necessary. If you must move on, leave a note where you first realize you are lost. Record the day and time you arrived, when you left, and in which direction you've gone. If you can't find a scrap of paper, scratch a message on a piece of bark or leave a piece of brightly colored fabric in the most visible spot you can find.

SIGNALING FOR HELP

Find a hilltop or a clearing in woods. If you have the means and it is safe to do so, build a fire. During the day, use green wood, leaves, grass—anything damp enough to smolder and produce lots of smoke. At night use dry material to make a bright, clear flame, taking care to keep it under control.

A series of three signals is a universal call of distress. Three whistle blasts or gunshots may work if anybody is near enough to hear. Remember that wind and flowing water will usually drown out the sound of a human voice, so don't waste energy yelling. Three big piles of dark-colored brush or rocks on snow or sand, or three piles of light-colored rock or other light-colored material against a dark background, are good signals. A group of three fires is great as long as you can maintain control of them. Spread out any brightly colored gear, tents, tarps, clothing, and Mylar space blankets that will be noticeable from the air. If you have the time, space, and energy, a giant SOS, or even a big X on the ground might attract attention.

A signal mirror is lightweight, easy to carry, and simple to use if you first practice aiming it. If your compass has a mirror, you can use that, too, but not as effectively. A true signaling mirror is shiny on both sides and has a hole in the middle. Hold it a couple of feet in front of you and point the hole toward your target (say a passing plane). To signal distress, give three flashes by passing your hand between the mirror and your target three times. (See illustration on page 30.)

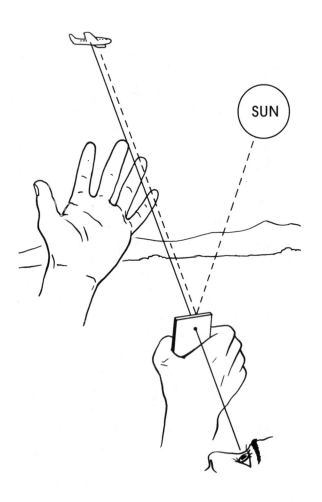

Using a signal mirror

If the only mirror you have is the one on your compass or a cosmetic mirror, it's worth using, though it isn't as easy to aim. Hold the shiny side toward the target as before. Extend your other arm out full length toward the target, with your fingers pointing up, and sight the target right over the longest finger. Then turn the mirror to catch the sunlight so it reflects a sunspot on your finger, and tilt it up just a bit so the spot points at the target.

Obviously, this won't work on a cloudy day.

Survival Priorities and First Aid

PRIORITIES

Most wilderness survival situations are resolved within twenty-four to forty-eight hours. Statistically, you'll find your own way to safety or will be rescued by others or you won't. Knowledge of what to do first is critical.

Your first priority, of course, is to tend to any immediate, life-threatening injuries, such as lack of breathing or heartbeat, loss of consciousness, profuse bleeding, broken bones, spinal injury, and shock. For specific information on dealing with wilderness first-aid situations, consult the FalconGuide *Wilderness First Aid*.

The following chapters discuss very rough approximations of what comes next, but the information may help direct your energies most efficiently in a crisis.

You can survive:

- Three to five hours without shelter from the cold.

- Three to five days without water.

- Three to five weeks without food.

Of course a person immersed in icy water can die in minutes, and one can become fatally dehydrated in less than a day in the desert in summertime. On the other hand, people have been known to endure fasts of many weeks and survive. The survival priorities are meant to remind you not to waste valuable time, sweat, and energy and to get yourself and your companions warm, dry, and out of the wind before night falls.

FIRST AID

There's no 911 in the wilderness.

While everyone should have basic first-aid skills, those who spend much time in the wilderness need to go a step further. First aid, by definition, is the aid you give to keep a sick or injured person alive and stable until professional medical help arrives. In the wilderness, however, professional medical help is not going to reach you for a long time, if at all.

In addition to basic first aid in the wilderness, you need to know when, where, and how to send for help, if there is any; when to evacuate a victim, if possible; and how to do it safely. You need to be aware of the problems peculiar to the wilderness, such as snakebite, high-altitude reactions, and lightning. You must know how to recognize and treat hypothermia and frostbite, heat exhaustion, and heat stroke. Covering all of these topics is not within the scope of this book, although knowledge of them is necessary for survival in the wilderness. All first-aid situations can turn into survival situations even after first aid is administered.

There are many good books available on mountaineering and wilderness medicine. Study at home and carry a compact edition such as *Wilderness First Aid* with you on wilderness outings. Better yet, get some hands-on training. Many organizations, including the Sierra Club, the Mountaineers, Wilderness Medicine Outfitters, and the Wilderness Medical Society, offer or can direct you to courses on backcountry medical skills.

Shelter from Cold and Heat

Should you become involved in a wilderness emergency, you are statistically much more likely to succumb to hypothermia, otherwise known as exposure, than to any other problem. If you can stay warm enough to make it through the first night, you're probably going to make it to safety or at least survive long enough to be rescued.

THE RECIPE FOR HYPOTHERMIA

The recipe for hypothermia has three ingredients: cold, wetness, and wind, so they are the conditions to avoid:

• **Cold.** If that sounds pretty obvious, note that most cases of hypothermia occur at 30 to 50 degrees Farenheit, when you're less likely to feel uncomfortable and do something about it until it's too late. In the afternoon sunshine it's easy to forget that temperatures can drop very dramatically at night, especially in deserts and at high elevations.

• **Wet.** Water conducts heat 240 times faster than still air. That means that when you're wet, you can lose body heat as much as 240 times faster than when you're dry. Remember, too, that sweat is just as wet as rain or melting snow.

• **Wind.** Your body constantly produces heat and radiates it out into the air, but even a gentle breeze on bare skin has plenty of cooling power, and the faster the wind blows, the colder you become. That's wind-chill, and it's especially deadly when skin or clothing is wet.

Planning Ahead

It is easier to stay warm than to get warm. As soon as you get into camp (assuming you have a camp) change your clothes (if you have any to change), especially if you've been sweating during the day, and more especially if you've been wearing an absorbent fabric such as cotton. At least one garment made of either wool or a synthetic wicking material such as polypropylene should always be with you. (See "Proper Clothing," page 41.)

Table 1: WINDCHILL

Air temperature (°F)	Wind speed in miles per hour								
	0	5	10	15	20	25	30	35	40
	Equivalent windchill temperature								
35	35	32	22	16	12	8	6	4	3
30	30	27	16	9	4	1	-2	-4	-5
25	25	22	10	2	-3	-7	-10	-12	-13
20	20	16	3	-5	-10	-15	-18	-20	-21
15	15	11	-3	-11	-17	-22	-25	-27	-29
10	10	6	-9	-18	-24	-29	-33	-35	-37
5	5	0	-15	-25	-31	-36	-41	-43	-45
0	0	-5	-22	-31	-39	-44	-49	-52	-53
-5	-5	-10	-27	-38	-46	-51	-56	-58	-60
-10	-10	-15	-34	-45	-53	-59	-64	-67	-69
-15	-15	-21	-40	-51	-60	-66	-71	-74	-76
-20	-20	-26	-46	-58	-67	-74	-79	-82	-84
-25	-25	-31	-52	-65	-74	-81	-86	-89	-92

Shaded area indicates high risk of cold-related injuries.

Under normal camping conditions, it's always wise to warm up thoroughly by the campfire and/or have a hot drink just before you jump into your sleeping bag. Don't wait until you're already cold or you'll spend half the night building up enough body heat to allow the bag to do its job. Your sleeping bag can't create heat; it can only preserve yours.

Recognizing Hypothermia

Hypothermia is defined as loss of core body temperature. Your core is inside your torso, where all those vital organs are. When you become critically cold, your body is willing to sacrifice fingers and toes in favor of saving the whole organism, so your blood leaves the extremities and rushes to the center, leaving you subject to frostbite. (More about frostbite later.)

Hypothermia claims so many victims because it can sneak up slowly, then pounce so hard and fast nobody realizes there's anything amiss until it's too late. Your body can operate only within a narrow range of internal temperatures. At 90 degrees it can no longer warm itself by any of the mechanisms designed for that purpose, such as shivering, and unless heat is added from some outside source the temperature continues to fall until, at somewhere around 80 degrees, you slip into a coma and die. The danger of hypothermia is one of the most important reasons for hiking in the wilderness with a companion.

An early sign of hypothermia is violent, uncontrolled shivering. That's one way the body produces heat. Shivering can be so intense that it becomes almost impossible to do the simple things that need to be done to warm up, such as zipping zippers, snapping snaps, or lighting matches. If you don't manage to stop losing heat immediately, you begin to stumble; your body becomes so rigid that you cease to shiver. Speech becomes difficult; your mouth won't cooperate, and even if you could speak, you probably wouldn't make any sense, because by then, your mental processes aren't functioning either.

Wilderness travelers must be alert to changes in their companions' behavior. An uncharacteristic lack of enthusiasm, depression, lethargy, disorientation, or confusion that otherwise can't be explained is cause for concern. The most experienced person is as much at risk as the beginner because memory and judgment may fail. The victim often denies feeling cold and may insist through chattering teeth and with fumbling fingers that everything is just fine. Victims sometimes refuse the offer of more warm clothing or stand shivering in the wind clutching a warm parka without putting it on. If you travel alone, you simply must be prepared for cold, and you must take care of yourself at the very first sign of a chill.

Treating Hypothermia

First, prevent any further heat loss. If it's windy or wet, get the victim out of the wind and out of all wet clothing, right down to the skin. Then dry the person's hair if possible and put him or her into dry clothing and a sleeping bag. If the person is in very serious condition, you may need to prewarm a sleeping bag with your own or someone else's body heat, or crawl right in with the victim and share your own internal furnace (as long as you're not wet, too). If the person is conscious, a hot drink will warm the core. (Remember never to give liquids to an unconscious victim. If the fluid goes into the lungs instead of the stomach, the victim will drown.) Hypothermia victims often feel drowsy, but keep them awake until you're sure they're out of danger, especially if they've been shivering. Shivering helps keep them warm, and they'll probably stop if they fall asleep.

Never, never drink alcohol when the weather is very cold, and never give it to a hypothermia victim. Liquor expands the capillaries near the surface of the skin, pulling blood and warmth from the body core where it's needed. It's especially dangerous because it makes you feel warm enough that you're less likely to dress properly or otherwise take care of yourself.

FROSTBITE

Frostbite occurs when blood flow to fingers, toes, nose, and cheeks is reduced, allowing the tissues in these extremities to freeze. Frostbitten skin looks colorless and waxy, but because all sensation in the affected area is lost, the victim is often unaware of the problem. If not treated quickly, fingers and toes may be lost to gangrene. Treat by tucking the affected part into an armpit or other warm cranny or by immersing in warm water. Don't rub the skin vigorously or you'll further damage the fragile tissue. Prevent frostbite by layering your clothing (see "Proper Clothing" below), by consuming a steady and adequate flow of fluids, and by avoiding excess sweating.

PROPER CLOTHING

Your first line of defense against cold is, of course, your clothing, and the most efficient way of dressing for the wilderness is layering. Clothing protects by holding a thin layer of air, warmed by body heat, close to the body; the more layers, the more heat retained. Several light layers are better than one heavy jacket or parka.

Layering also allows you to more finely tune your comfort level by peeling off or adding just enough. Too much heat is as dangerous as too little in cold weather, since you need to avoid sweating.

Know how to tell the outdoor novices from the veterans at a glance? The novices are wearing jeans. Jeans are sturdy and tough and all-American, but they are inappropriate and downright dangerous if the weather turns bad. Like any cotton fabric, they absorb water and hold it. (That's why towels are made of cotton.) When jeans are wet, they're heavy and take forever to dry. Cotton T-shirts and sweatshirts have the same drawbacks. If you must wear cotton, make sure you have other clothing to change into.

It may seem paradoxical, but you'll get along in nature more comfortably and safely with many of the new synthetic fabrics. The best are made of various polyester filaments or other high-tech material and are designed to shed moisture, to wick water away from your skin, to provide insulation even when wet, and to dry very quickly. The only natural material to keep you warm even when it's wet is wool, but it's heavy, especially when it's wet, it dries very slowly, and some people find it much too itchy. The synthetic materials are designed to be worn next to the skin so they

---

If your feet get cold, put on a hat.

---

can wick away body moisture. Over these go a heavier polypro or wool garment. If it's very cold, add a heavy pile, fleece, or down layer. Then top it all with a windproof/waterproof shell.

The part of you that requires at least as much and perhaps even more blood than your body core is your brain. That keeps everything, including all your internal organs, running. At least half of your body's heat is lost through your head, which is why humans have hair up there (at least some do), but human hair does not insulate all that well. The most important article of clothing in your outdoor wardrobe is a warm hat. Warm gloves or mittens and warm socks are wonderful inventions, but if your head and torso are warm, hands and feet are better able to take care of themselves.

Don't venture far from civilization without some kind of wind and rain protection, no matter what the weather looks like in the morning. A typical summer day in the Rockies, the Sierra Nevada, or the Himalayas, and even some of our Southwestern deserts, often begins with bright sunshine against a deep blue sky followed by a few wisps of cloud drifting innocently in around noon, and then angry black thunderheads, howling winds, driving rain, hail, or even snow by midafternoon. The temperature may fall as much as 60 degrees in an hour. This is *not* a rare or unusual occurrence. This is normal mountain weather; don't be bluffed into leaving your rain gear in the car. Sometimes by dark, the sky is clear and full of stars again, but there's a good chance that if you're caught unprepared, night will fall before you have a chance to dry out and warm up again, and then you're in trouble. Worse yet, there's always the possibility that Mother Nature is really mad and has sent in a weather front that will rage for days on end.

Table 2: PROPER CLOTHING

Top (torso, from skin layer out)	Bottom (legs)
Lightweight polypro long underwear	Lightweight polypro long underwear
Midweight polypro or wool sweater	Fast-drying long pants
Fleece, pile, or down jacket	
Wind/rain jacket with hood	Wind/rain pants

Also include a wood or fleece hat, gloves, and wool socks.

Ideally you'll always have with you a windproof, waterproof, breathable Gore-Tex or other superfabric rain parka with hood and armpit vents, matching rain pants, and all sorts of Velcro doodads, but a coated nylon jacket will do. Ponchos are popular and inexpensive and can double as overhead tarps or ground sheets, but they let the rain in when they flap in the wind and are dangerous to hike in since you can't see your feet or the ground just ahead. At the very least, carry a couple of large trash bags, thirty-gallon size or larger. They can be folded into a tiny package, stowed in a corner of a daypack or in a pocket, and can be used for a rain suit (cut a hole in the top for your head), an emergency pack cover (cut two slits up the back for the shoulder straps), and countless other purposes.

Table 2 (see above) gives a summary of proper clothing layers.

What If You Don't Have Proper Clothing?

Should you find yourself in a survival situation without enough insulation, you can improvise by stuffing almost anything you can find that's dry into whatever you are wearing. Street people in cities know about lining their clothes with newspaper. You can stuff a map, leaves, or pine needles between two layers of clothing to provide dead-air spaces to trap body heat. You can use the wonderful soft insulating fluff that cattails, willows, milkweed, and other plants produce to disperse their seeds, but you can't always count on finding yourself in trouble near a cattail patch at just the right time of year.

FINDING SHELTER

If you're an alert outdoorsperson, you will have noticed that sometimes as you round a corner or descend into a ferny little creekbed you feel a very distinct difference in temperature. These little pockets of warmth or cold are microclimates. You need to be aware of them when you're searching for the coziest spot to spend the night. Here are some hints:

• *Camp on the south-facing slope.* If you're in hilly or mountainous country (and if you're in the Northern Hemisphere), south-facing slopes are warmer and drier than north-facing ones since they get more sun during the day. You don't need a compass to tell the difference, and if you're paying attention, you don't even need to see the sun. The vegetation on the south-facing slope is usually lighter in color and lower and shrubbier in texture because the plants that grow there don't have to produce as much chlorophyll to feed themselves as their north-facing neighbors do.

• *Camp partway up a hillside rather than on a ridgetop or in a bowl or valley.* Ridgetops are exposed to the wind, and cold air tends to sink and pool in low places. The difference in temperature between a river valley and a terrace 50 feet upslope may be as much as 20 degrees.

• *Camp downhill from a stable wind blocker such as a big rock or a downed log.* Make sure the object is stable before using it for wind protection. Cold air flows uphill during the daytime and downhill at night, so take advantage of any natural windbreak.

• *Avoid gullies.* Don't camp in places that look like runoff routes for water. Also be wary of bowl-shaped tent sites.

◗ Survival Technique: LEAN-TO SHELTER

If you have time to pile up a debris hut or some kind of lean-to shelter, by all means do what you can to ensure your safety and comfort for the night, but beware of soaking yourself in sweat or burning up vital stores of energy in order to create some outdoor architectural marvel. Your goals are to stay dry and conserve body heat.

A simple and efficient shelter is a large downed log, with a series of branches propped against it, covered with brush or leafy branches. If you have a tarp or a plastic trash bag to stretch over the supports before piling on the brush, so much the better. Build a small fire at the head end, but not too close.

It is not true that moss always grows on the north side of the tree.

Since heat rises, including the heat produced by your body, the most critical part of any shelter is the roof. Burrowing down next to the trunk of a tree with low overhanging branches will provide good protection in wooded country.

Another important requirement will be insulation between your body and the cold earth. At 98.6 degrees Farenheit you will lose heat to any surface that's colder than you are. Any extra clothing, bark, twigs, leaves, or pine needles between you and the ground will work if they're dry. Trash bags make it easy to collect insulating material, and when stuffed with pine needles they make very comfy mattresses.

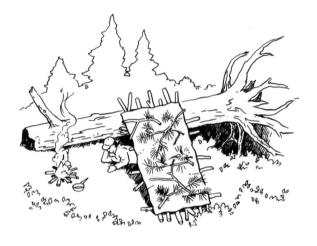

Lean-to shelter

Snow is an excellent form of insulation. It blocks out wind and traps and reflects your body heat. Snow caves are fun to build and comfortable to sleep in, but if you're in the middle of a survival situation, you may not have the time or energy to build one. You can, however, dig out a trench just large enough to fit your body and spread branches, or even your pack or boat, over the top for a roof.

Caution: Make sure the branches you use are substantial enough to support a heavy snow load without collapsing and that they are long enough to extend at least a foot on either side of the trench.

Forest trees often have wells around their trunks where snow has not accumulated very deeply, and sometimes not at all, because of the protection of over-hanging branches and because the dark-colored bark

---

*Always carry extra trash bags
to keep yourself dry.*

---

absorbs heat and keeps snow melted. These are wonderful emergency shelters that require almost no preparation at all, but you must have some kind of waterproof material between you and the walls. Your own heat will melt the surrounding snow, and your first concern is to keep dry, no matter what! A trash bag or two and a few branches to keep you out of direct contact with the snow may save your life.

If you're lucky enough to find yourself near some overhanging rocks or caves, take advantage of them. Pick a place that's large enough so you won't have to touch the walls and lose heat by conduction but small enough to hold in your body heat. It is a good idea before you crawl in to make sure your bedroom isn't already occupied by something furry or slithery.

Once you're tucked in, keep plenty of food and water nearby if you have it, and nibble and drink frequently. Staying fully hydrated helps keep you warm. Think of water as a form of antifreeze that keeps your blood circulating freely so it can warm you efficiently. Even if you have to urinate during the night, it will be worth it. Occasional handfuls of high-energy, sugary food—trail mix, dried fruit, granola, even candy—will provide you with a ready source of fuel for your body to burn.

If you're still not warm enough, try doing isometric exercises, tensing and relaxing groups of muscles, but don't work out so vigorously that you work up a sweat, burn valuable energy too fast, or puff and pant, breathing out warm internal air, and letting in cold outside air. Shivering is itself an involuntary form of exercise and can raise body temperature significantly. Don't fight it.

⬇ *Survival Technique:*
COLD WATER SURVIVAL POSITION

Cold water draws away body warmth much faster than cold air does. If you fall into an ocean or a lake, and you have doubts about your ability to swim to shore, or if you're with companions or a rescue is possible, you may be able to survive for thirty to sixty minutes, depending on the water temperature.

Your priority is to keep yourself warm enough to retain consciousness until help arrives. Vigorous activity burns calories, so don't try to swim; conserve energy. Don't remove your clothes, but if you have any insulating material at hand, cover your head with it since

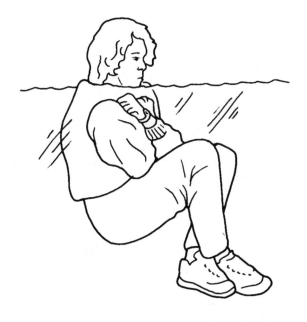

Cold water survival position

that's where you lose heat fastest. Draw your arms and legs in toward your chest and torso and hug yourself to hold in your core body heat. If several people are in the water together, huddle to share body warmth.

This of course is only a short-term survival technique and should be used only if you have a chance of rescue in a short time. Otherwise, it is advisable to do your best to swim to shore. Once at shore, follow survival practices discussed in this chapter and build a fire.

STAYING COOL

Finding shelter from heat is a bigger challenge than finding shelter from the cold, since your body constantly produces heat on its own. Still, there are steps you can take to protect yourself from the external environment when it is even hotter than you are.

• Stay in the shade whenever possible.

• Wear loose-fitting clothing that covers as much of your body as possible to prevent sunburn and so that sweat is not evaporated so fast that it's wasted.

• Wear a hat to keep the sun from beating directly on your head, heating the dense concentration of blood vessels there.

• Where there is no shade, avoid sitting directly on the ground. Ground temperature may be 30 degrees hotter than the air even 12 inches above it. Sit on a rock, your pack, or a pile of clothing.

Starting an Emergency Fire

FIRE-MAKING BASICS

The campfire is the symbol of outdoor life, yet more than one-quarter of wilderness users don't know how to build one or keep it lit. Stranger still, search-and-rescue teams report that many victims of hypothermia and related problems never even try.

In recent years many national parks and other wilderness areas have prohibited campfires in areas that get heavy use, in order to protect fragile ecosystems, and near or above timberline. Backpackers and others are required to use portable stoves for cooking and are expected to dress warmly enough to camp comfortably without a fire. Still, in a life-or-death emergency, fire making is a skill everybody needs to have. (If you need more motivation, read Jack London's short story "To Build a Fire.")

Murphy's Law seems to operate with a vengeance whenever you really need a fire. The more urgent your need, the wetter the tinder, the more violent the wind, the fouler the language. A systematic, step-by-step approach works best, along with the knowledge that a fire needs only three elements: fuel, oxygen, and a spark.

First, clear a small area—a reasonable distance from trees or logs or overhanging branches—of any burnable material, sweeping away everything right down to mineral soil or rock. Next, note wind direction.

Regardless of local policy on fire,
fire-making is always legal
in a life-or-death emergency.

Build a ring of bare soil or rocks to contain your fire, and make sure it's higher and tighter on the windward side.

Assemble all your fire-making materials next. You'll need several sizes of tinder and kindling within easy reach before you begin, or your tinder may burn itself out while you're off gathering bigger pieces and you'll have to start over.

Start with the finest tinder possible. Almost all novices try to light sticks that are way too big. Fine, dry, stringy material is best; dried grasses, finely shredded but not powdered, and juniper bark are excellent.

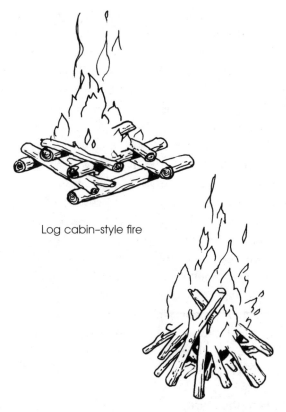

Log cabin–style fire

Tepee–style fire

Whittle larger sticks into smaller sticks and use the shavings for tinder. Best of all is light, dry, fluffy plant material such as milkweed or cattail fluff, goats-beard lichen, or potato chips. Clothes-dryer lint works beautifully if you happen to have any. Next assemble a pile of slightly coarser stuff: pine needles, very small twigs, nothing bigger in diameter than a wooden match. In wet weather, a great place to find such material is near the base of a tree where dense foliage down low on the trunk shields the ground from rain or snow-fall. Then progress to pencil-size pieces, and so on.

Pile these materials loosely in either a tepee or log-cabin shape so that individual twigs are close enough together to spread the flame from one to another, but with plenty of space between them for air to circulate. Make sure the finer material has a good start before piling on heavier pieces or you'll suffocate your fire.

A very common error is building too big a blaze. There's no need to wear yourself out or work up a sweat collecting mountains of firewood. You can huddle closer to a smaller fire and stay more comfortable than at a larger one, where you can easily scorch your back-side while your front side freezes.

Striking the Spark

There are all kinds of clever gimmicks on the market for starting a flame, but none so reliable as a dry match. You can store books of matches inside zippered plastic bags, watertight pill bottles, or film canisters any place: in your pocket, backpack, tackle box, or any nook or cranny. You can also buy windproof and waterproof matches at outfitting stores, but they won't light just anywhere. They require a striker, and the striker must be kept dry to work. Disposable lighters are wonderful inventions, too, but they're not foolproof. Always carry a few matches as backup.

There are any number of fire-making devices you can make from natural materials: bow drills, hand drills, flint and steel, and more, and these are effective and satisfying to make and to learn to use. In a real emergency, however, where time is of the essence, all the materials will have to be assembled, all require some kind of tool, at least a pocket knife, and all require plenty of skill and practice. If the idea appeals to you, you can make a bow drill or other device, learn to use it at home, and carry it with you on your outdoor expeditions, but a simple book of matches (or several) is best.

Caution: Do not splash stove fuel all over everything and throw in a match. The fuel will flare all at once, singe everybody's eyebrows, burn away completely, and leave you with nothing. If you're in a serious survival situation, you have enough problems without having to deal with severe burns.

○ *Survival Technique:*
THE BOW DRILL

You will need the following:

• **Fire board.** A flat piece of wood at least 18 inches long and about ½ inch thick, made of a relatively soft wood such as cottonwood. Drill a hole about an inch from the edge of the board, then whittle out a triangular notch from the edge of the board to the hole.

• **Drill.** A rounded, foot-long stick, slightly pointed at the top end, rounder at the bottom. It can be made of the same wood as the board.

• **Socket.** A hand-size piece of very hard wood, or even a stone, with a depression deep enough to hold the top of the drill steady while it's spun.

• **Bow.** A smooth branch about 2 feet long, limber enough not to crack but not too flexible. The bowstring can be made of natural cordage material or a piece of rawhide, such as a bootlace, twisted until just before it kinks. Attach the string to the ends of the bow, just tightly enough so that you can make a tight loop around the drill.

Now prepare a little nest of fine tinder and arrange it so that it lies directly under the notch in the fire board. Hold down the end of the board with one foot. Wind the bowstring one complete turn around the

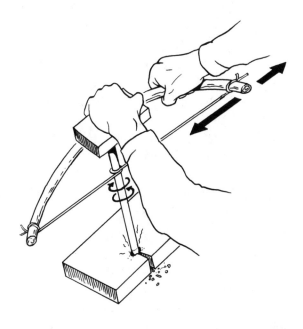

Bow drill

drill and insert the rounded end of the drill into the hole in the board. Hold it in the socket and draw the bow back and forth quickly and smoothly (a steady rhythm is more important than extreme speed) until the friction on the fire board causes smoke to rise and hot embers to trickle down the notch into your nest of tinder.

Soon the friction will produce a spark that will fall onto the tinder. As soon as that happens, remove the board and gently fan or blow the spark into flame.

Another excellent but simple bit of equipment is a little stub of a candle or some commercial fire starter, which comes in small tubes or small bricks. You have to light either with a match, but they will give you a flame that lasts longer, possibly enough longer to coax slightly damp tinder into flame.

◯ Survival Technique:
MAKING A FIRE BED

This is the coziest possible way to spend the night in the wilderness without shelter, but it takes several hours and plenty of energy to prepare, so this method is practical only if you know there's plenty of daylight left and that there's no possibility of rescue for another day or two.

For one person, if time and energy are running out, the minimum dimensions for your bed are 1 foot by 3 feet, though you can dig a trench the length and width of your whole body for extra comfort. The important dimension is the depth. It should be as close to 8 inches as you can make it. If the hole is deeper, you might not stay warm enough and will have wasted energy. If it's too shallow, the bed will be too warm to sleep on, and might even burn you.

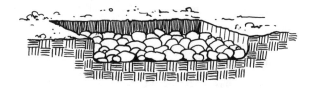

Stones laid for the fire bed

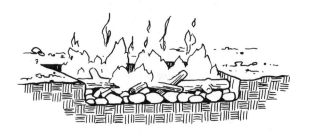

Fire burning on top of the stones

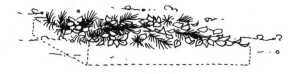

Fire bed covered with dirt, then dry vegetation

Dig the trench, then line the bottom with rocks about 2½ inches in diameter. Arrange them in a flat mosaic, as close to one another as possible. Then add wood and burn a hot fire on top of the rocks for a couple of hours.

When it has burned down, refill the hole with the dirt you originally removed and pack it down. Refill it *completely*. If the layer of dirt covering the hot rocks is too thin, you'll roast.

Let the bed stand for another couple of hours, if you have time, to allow the moisture in the soil to steam away. Otherwise, you'll need to sleep with a tarp or plastic trash bags beneath you to avoid waking up soaked to the skin. For real luxury, make a mattress by covering the bed with several inches of pine needles or leaves.

If you prop some leafy branches or can rig a piece of plastic or other material over the top half of your body, so that the heat rising from the fire bed will be reflected back down upon you, you'll be warm and cozy even in severe weather. Heat will continue to rise from the bed for a second night.

Caution: Be very careful where you locate your fire bed. Make sure you're out of the way of any overhanging tree or anything flammable. Remove any roots you encounter underground as you dig. They can ignite and smolder for a day and then start a forest fire.

Water Emergencies

The body is about 75 percent water and doesn't function very long or very well on any less. If you allow your reserves to become just one or two quarts low (equal to two to four pounds of body weight) your ability to function will be reduced by a full 25 percent. In a survival situation, you're likely not to be at your physical peak, and giving yourself a further handicap could be fatal.

Dehydration is sneaky. You can sweat more than one quart every hour when you're working hard in hot weather. Don't assume you're not losing fluids just because you're not dripping with sweat. When the air is dry and cold, perspiration can evaporate before it reaches the skin surface where you can feel it. Puffing and panting open-mouthed with exertion releases lots of moisture, too. When you notice your breath on a cold day, you're seeing condensing water. The harder you breathe, the more you lose. All the functions your body performs to maintain itself, even while you're asleep—breathing, digesting, regulating temperature—

use water. If you've ever spent the night in a poorly ventilated tent, you likely awoke to find the walls and ceiling dripping into little puddles along the sides. That water came from you.

YOUR SENSE OF THIRST

By the time your mouth is dry and you're craving a drink, it's going to be hard to catch up on the water you need. Think back to the last time you needed to water some trailside bushes. If you're not urinating as frequently as usual, or if your urine is dark in color, you're dehydrated. Be aware that symptoms that may be attributed to other causes such as altitude sickness or even flu can be signs of dehydration. Headache, dizziness, nausea, and cramps often disappear like magic with just a little rest and lots of water. Don't ignore such symptoms; they may be early signs of more serious, even deadly conditions such as heat exhaustion and heat stroke.

Fortunately, even though the consequences are serious, prevention and treatment of dehydration are simple as long as water is available: *drink, drink, and drink!* If it helps, set your watch to remind yourself to drink at twenty-minute intervals, and do it, thirsty or not. Tank up before you set out in the morning and last thing at night. Drink every time you think about it.

You cannot train or condition yourself to survive on less water. The military has considered that this would be a valuable ability for soldiers to learn in desert campaigns, but they found that it cannot be done. You can, however, acclimate yourself to hot weather. Studies have shown that it takes about ten days for the body to learn to cool itself more efficiently, and it does so by producing more perspiration. The better adjusted to hot weather you become, the more you need to drink.

When you're packing for an outing, overestimate the amount of water you'll need. As a rule, you'll use at least one gallon per day. If you're working strenuously or if the weather is hot, you'll need more. Carry water in two or more one-liter bottles instead of one big one in case you have a spill or spring a leak. Study maps to learn where to expect water sources, but don't rely on them. Springs shown on topographic maps may not be flowing in a dry year or late in the season.

There has been some recent discussion about the risk of hyponatremia—electrolyte imbalance brought about by drinking too much water. The symptoms are similar to those of dehydration, and the condition can be fatal. However, the chances of this becoming a problem for you in a wilderness emergency are very, very small. If the weather is hot, you are much more likely to suffer from too little rather than too much water. Carry some powdered electrolyte replacement drink with your ten essentials if you think you might be tempted to drink too much water.

RATION SWEAT, NOT WATER

If you have only a limited amount of water, drink it. It's of no use to you at all in your canteen or water bottle. Saving it for later is fruitless if you become too weak to signal for help or otherwise take care of yourself. Search-and-rescue people tell too many stories about the number of victims they have encountered who have died of thirst with full canteens at their sides.

Suggestions for rationing sweat:

• Travel at night or in the morning when it's cooler.

• Wear loose-fitting clothing that covers as much of your body as possible so that sweat is not evaporated so fast that it's wasted, and to prevent sunburn.

• Wear a hat to keep the sun from beating directly on your head, heating the dense concentration of blood vessels there.

• Where there is no shade, avoid sitting directly on the ground. Ground temperature may be 30 degrees hotter than the air even 12 inches above it. Sit on a rock, your pack, or a pile of clothing.

• Avoid alcohol, coffee, black tea, cola drinks—anything with alcohol or caffeine. These diuretics draw water from your tissues where it's needed. You may long for a cold beer, but it's the last thing you need unless you have plenty of water to dilute it.

• Avoid food. Digestion takes lots of water, so if there's no water to drink, don't eat. High-protein foods require more water to digest than carbohydrates do. Odd as it may seem, a dry cracker is less dehydrating than a juicy piece of meat.

Store water in your stomach not your canteen.

• Avoid salt tablets. They're likely to make you sick, especially if you don't wash them down with lots of water. They usually consist of nothing but sodium chloride, while you'll also be losing other important salts such as potassium. Furthermore, when your body becomes acclimated to hot weather—that is, when you've been exercising in hot weather for a week or so—it retains the salts it needs instead of releasing them into perspiration. If you're in good condition, don't worry about adding extra salt to your diet.

FINDING WATER

If you find yourself in a survival situation without water, stop and do a little mental calculation before taking any action. Remember that any expenditure of energy uses water. If there's a good chance of rescue by day's end, and if it's very hot, keep still and wait. If on the other hand you think you might be in for a long ordeal and are feeling strong, seeking water or constructing some device to gather it might be worthwhile.

All living things need water. The air and the very earth itself can yield up moisture even in arid regions, if you know what to do.

Try to find some high ground where you can scan the landscape. If the area is mountainous, check north-facing slopes first; they usually receive more precipitation, get less sunlight, and are wetter. Note channels where water has run before. Are there any darker patches that might indicate dampness? Look for low points where water might collect. Be alert for changes in vegetation; a patch or a line of darker green against the usual gray-green of desert scrub or sagebrush could lead you to a spring. Examine canyon walls or cliff-sides for changes in color that might be water stains, especially where two different rock strata meet. At these places, water is often forced to the surface in a line of seeps and springs, which often support hanging gardens or patches of moss that make them visible from a distance.

Learn to identify a few of the more common and widespread plants that send roots downward to tap shallow sources of groundwater. Willows, cottonwoods, sedges, rushes, and cattails are very reliable indicators of accessible water. (There are plenty of good field guides and knowledgeable people to help you learn to recognize them.) All you have to do when you spot some of these is dig. If you're lucky, just a few inches will be enough. You might have to dig a basin and wait until water seeps in to fill it from below, or even press out moisture from damp soil with a bandana or T-shirt.

Water often flows underground even where there is no plant life. Find a streambed whose bottom isn't made of fine deep sand and dig down a foot or two. If there is no indication of dampness by that depth, give up and try somewhere else.

Dew is another possible source of moisture, even in deserts. In the very early morning when the air is still, it condenses on plants and rocks and other smooth surfaces, including plastic and metal. Spread out one of those indispensable trash bags at night to catch some. You can sop it up with your bandana or T-shirt and wring it into your mouth.

In rocky areas you may find depressions ranging from the size of teacups to deep ponds that collect rainwater. These are called "tanks" or *tinajas* in the West, and the larger ones, sometimes shaded by surrounding rocks, may hold water year-round. If you find one of these oases, take what you need and go away, if possible. Never camp near one of these pools if you can help it. Desert animals such as bighorn sheep depend on these water sources and may die if frightened away from their waterholes by humans.

While it is not safe to depend on animals to show you what to eat, their behavior may give you hints about where to find water. Grazing animals, such as the range cattle ubiquitous throughout the West, moving purposefully in one direction, especially in the morning and evening, are often going to water. When they've had enough, their grazing movements become more random and aimless. If there is one path that seems to be more heavily used than others, there's a good chance it leads to water. It might be a muddy old stock tank, green with cow slobber, but it could save your life. Don't waste your time watching rodents. Many desert critters, such as kangaroo rats, have special metabolisms that allow them to live their entire lives without drinking!

Back to that scummy stock tank or pothole. You know it's seething with bacteria and is bound to wreak havoc with your insides. If you have no way to purify it, should you drink it or not? If your situation is truly desperate, and there is no water but dirty water, drink it. Consider the odds: If you drink nothing, you're going to die for sure. If you drink polluted water you may or may not get sick, and one way or another you'll buy yourself some time. If you do get sick, it probably won't become debilitating for a day or more. If the microorganism in question is *Giardia lamblia,* the most common backcountry culprit, you won't get any symptoms for at least a week, by which time you could be safe and sound and under medical care. (More about treating water later.)

WATER MYTHS
• Should I cut down a cactus?

Remember those old cowboy movies where the hero hacks off the top of a cactus and scoops out the clear, cool water with his ten-gallon hat? That only happens in Hollywood. Cacti do store lots of moisture, but they protect it very well with thick, tough skins and long, sharp spines. The average pocketknife isn't nearly long enough to penetrate a big one, and even if you have a machete, what you'll find inside is not a clear pool but a stringy, dense pulp. You might be able to squeeze some moisture out of this, and it is sometimes drinkable, but much more often it's bitter and unpalatable and is likely to cause nausea or vomiting, the last thing you need in an emergency.

• Should I drink urine?

Another popular myth is that you can survive by drinking urine or even blood. Those who have done so and lived have survived in spite of their actions, not because of them. Your urinary system is designed to collect all kinds of nasty toxic substances your body needs to get rid of, to mix them with water, and to flush them out. Drinking urine amounts to deliberately reintroducing all those toxins into your system so that your body will need more water to get rid of them.

- **Should I eat snow?**

You don't usually think of thirst as a problem when there's snow on the ground, but the water contained in snow is not in a form your body can use. Do not eat snow in a wilderness emergency. Shoveling cold snow into your warm insides, lowering your core body temperature, is inviting hypothermia, but there's a more critical objection. You can't pack your tissues and bloodstream with snow; they can only absorb water in liquid form. When you eat snow, your body must expend lots of energy to melt it, which in turn requires lots of water that has to come from those same tissues and you end up more dehydrated.

MAKING DRINKABLE WATER

Drinkable water can be made from both snow and polluted water. It can also be distilled from urine, plant material, or the soil itself, but this requires some basic equipment, plenty of time, and lots of energy.

Water from Snow

If you have a stove and adequate fuel or have fire-making material and a pot, and wind and weather conditions aren't too horrible, by all means, melt some snow. Do remember to put at least a half inch of water in the bottom of the pot first, though, before you add the snow. If you put a container of snow directly over a flame, the snow will evaporate before it melts and you'll be left with a scorched and empty pot. Snow takes up much more volume than water does, so you'll need more than you think. If the snow is dry and powdery, it will take ten quarts of snow to produce a single quart of water.

If you don't have a stove or pot but can build a fire, gather a few stones, 4 to 5 inches in diameter, and put them in the fire for half an hour or so until they're very hot. Do not gather stones from a lake or riverbed: They can explode when heated too quickly. Scoop out a hole in the snow, at least 12 inches by 18 inches. Line the hole with a plastic trash bag. Refill the hole with loose snow, then toss in the hot rocks one at a time. The hot rocks will melt the snow in the hole and you can dip out the meltwater. Don't worry: The trash bag won't melt. You'll have water in minutes.

A plastic trash bag alone may be used to melt snow if there's even a hint of sunshine. Spread it out on a rock or some other surface with a depression in the middle to collect the water, and pile snow onto it. The dark color will absorb what heat there is and start the snow melting.

Treating Water

No matter how clear and sweet the water seems, backcountry water should be purified before drinking. Microbiologists from government agencies and universities by the dozens have sampled water from lakes and ponds, creeks and rivers, and have found that many sources harbor some kind of bug that can make you sick. Many of these organisms have been around for a long time but have become widespread only recently because of the increasing number of humans who have taken to the wilderness and have been careless about sanitation.

These organisms spread when somebody defecates in the woods and that material gets washed into water that somebody else drinks, or when people forget to wash their hands before sharing food or handling eating utensils. One of the most commonc culprits is *E. coli.* Another, *Giardia lamblia,* used to be known as "beaver fever," since these animals live most of their lives in water, but almost any mammal can carry the disease. Marmots, pikas, and rodents of all kinds can and do spread the parasite. So do domestic dogs.

Make sure you know what's upstream before you drink untreated water, and don't do it at all in areas where there are lots of people or cattle. If you're in a remote, unspoiled area, water near the surface of a lake is safer than water that is constantly stirred up in a rocky stream. Bacteria are vulnerable to UV light, and they get more concentrated and prolonged exposure in the relatively quiet water of a lake.

The good news is that diseases caused by these organisms are not fatal, though they may be unpleasant and debilitating. The usual symptoms include fatigue and weakness, loss of appetite, nausea, vomiting, cramps, gas, and diarrhea. Depending on the person, the dose, and the bug, you can get any, all, or none of these symptoms. Some of these diseases run their course and disappear in a day or two, others last a week, and still others go away and recur at intervals for years if untreated. Most are easily cured with antibiotics.

The bad news is that if you're in an emergency situation and are already weakened, exhausted, or dehydrated, a very few bouts of diarrhea or vomiting can be very serious indeed. Treat the water when you can.

Boiling kills all the bad bugs, but of course you must have the necessary container, stove, fuel, or firewood. Contrary to popular opinion, you do not have to maintain a hard rolling boil for ten minutes or more to kill any of the critters you'll find in North America. *Giardia,* for example, will die at temperatures far below boiling, so even at very high elevations where water boils at lower temperatures, just a few seconds at a hard boil is sufficient.

Iodine, in tablet form or in solution, should be a standard part of your survival kit (as long as you're not allergic). It will kill just about everything except *Cryptosporidium,* which is a bug that is beginning to show up in some water sources and causes non-life-threatening diarrhea. It's available at outfitting stores in the form of tablets or crystals, and some kinds can be purchased with a "chaser" chemical that kills the iodine taste after the iodine has killed the bugs. Follow the directions on the bottle carefully; if the water is very cold or very dirty, you'll need to use more iodine or let it stand longer. It's important to know, too, that iodine tablets (though not iodine crystals) lose their potency rapidly once the bottle has been opened. Don't save tablets from one year to the next.

There are dozens of filters available from wilderness outfitters that are lightweight (less than a pound) and inexpensive and will eliminate all protozoans and many bacteria. The smaller viruses can only be killed by chemical means (with iodine, for example) or by boiling. If you decide to use a filter, make sure the one you buy is guaranteed to remove *Giardia lamblia* and *Cryptosporidium*. Some filters contain purifiers that will also eliminate viruses, but these are heavier, more expensive, and clog quickly. Even if you own the fanciest filter or purifier on the market, keep some iodine tucked away in case the equipment breaks down. Any filter can clog, and you will still need to drink.

🔘 *Survival Technique:*
SOLAR STILL FOR MAKING WATER

This still will yield, at most, about a quart of water in twenty-four hours, so it is only worthwhile if you're planning to stay put for some time, happen to be carrying a clear plastic tarp and a water container, and can afford the sweat and energy needed to make it.

Dig a hole about 3 feet deep and 3 feet in diameter. Put an uncovered pot or other container in the center. If there are any green plants nearby, put them on the floor of the hole, too, to provide extra moisture. Spread a plastic tarp over the hole, then put a rock in the center of it, one big and heavy enough to pull the tarp downward to a point just above the water container. Cover the edges of the tarp very tightly with the dirt and rocks you removed from the hole. Make sure the sides of the tarp do not touch the inside walls of the hole. On a sunny day, moisture from the earth and from the plants you've added, if any, will condense on the underside of the tarp, flow down the slope, and drip off the point into the pot.

You can also use this method to distill clean water from urine or polluted water; just place the liquid in the bottom of the pit and position the tarp as above.

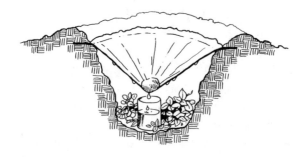

Solar still

Food Emergencies

THE LEAST OF YOUR WORRIES

Food has more value as a source of comfort and confidence than as a survival necessity. Odds are you'll get yourself out of your predicament, be rescued, or succumb to injury or cold long before you'll starve.

Most of us are used to eating at more or less regular intervals, and missing a few meals may be unpleasant but it won't be fatal. Fishing, snaring, trapping, or hunting require more time and energy than you'll probably have at your disposal in an emergency, even if you do have the necessary tools and skills. Concentrate instead on finding ways to conserve energy.

Still, becoming familiar with a few of the most widespread, nutritious, and easily recognizable wild food plants can go a long way toward making you feel at home in the wilderness. If you can collect enough food to provide you with calories to help you keep warm without burning even more energy finding and preparing it, do so. Many wildplants also produce useful material for insulation, fire starting, cordage making, or medicine.

It is important to keep in mind that there are no rules for distinguishing an edible from a poisonous

---

You should never eat a plant unless you can positively identify it as edible.

---

plant, so you must be able to positively identify each plant, to know which parts are edible, at what stage of growth it may be eaten, and how to prepare it. There are a great number of widely believed myths about wild plant foods.

EDIBLE PLANT MYTHS

• **It is safe to eat anything you observe other animals eating.**
False. Different animals have different digestive systems designed to accommodate different kinds of food. Ruminants—grazing animals such as cows—have four-chambered stomachs to enable them to digest the cellulose in grasses. Rodents and reindeer enjoy poisonous (to people) fly agaric mushrooms (Amanita muscaria).

• **All plants with white milky sap are poisonous.**
False. Some plants, such as the spurges, are toxic; others, such as the common dandelion, have been enjoyed for years; still others, such as milkweed, are poisonous when raw but delicious when cooked in three changes of boiling water.

• **A mushroom boiled in a pot with a silver coin will turn black if it's poisonous.**
False. It's unknown when or where this one originated, and anyway, when was the last time you saw a real silver coin?

• **A good test is to eat a tiny pinch of a plant, then wait. If you suffer no ill effects by the end of the day (or overnight), you can eat as much as you want.**
False. Some plants, fortunately very few, are deadly in very small quantities. Poison hemlock, water hemlock, and castor bean are good examples.

• **If it tastes good, it's safe to eat.**
False. Many victims who have survived amanita poisoning report that the mushrooms they ate were delicious.

A FEW WILD EDIBLE PLANTS

These are widespread and fairly easy to recognize, but consult field guides and/or experienced foragers to be sure of your identification before trying any of them.

Cattails

Those tall (up to 10 feet) dense stalks with grasslike leaves and a brown cigarlike structure toward the stem tip in summer inhabit wet marshy areas all over the world. Cattails are edible in some form or other year-round, even in winter when their aboveground parts have withered and died. The underground roots are white and crispy and delicious in any season once their Styrofoam-like covering has been scraped away. When they're only a few inches high in springtime, the young, colorless shoots of the new leaves are a crunchy addition to a salad. When the stalks have reached almost their full height, but before the cylindrical blooms appear, usually in late spring, feel along the stems for a fat pencil-size thickening near the top and peel the leaves away. Inside is the immature flower-to-be, and it can be eaten steamed or boiled like corn on the cob. When this part matures further, it becomes covered with generous handfuls of bright yellow pollen, which may be used as flour for baking breads, muffins, or pancakes.

Cattails have several valuable nonfood uses, too. In late summer when the flower cylinders have turned brown, fluffy, and soft, they can be shaken from the stems and stuffed between two layers of clothing as insulation. The brown flowers also make excellent tinder for fire starting. The leaves can be used for weaving.

Conifers

All cone-bearing trees (and occasionally shrubs) with needlelike leaves, such as pines, firs, and spruces, are conifers. Almost all conifers are evergreen and may be the only source of vitamin C when snow is on the ground. Just steep a handful of needles in hot water for a few minutes for a healthful tea.

Even the trunks of these trees conceal a source of food. Scrape or cut off the dry outer bark down to the moist tissue underneath. This is the cambium layer that conducts water and nutrients throughout the tree. It's tough and stringy but has been scraped out, chewed, or ground up as emergency food for centuries. Harvest this food only in an emergency, though. Damage to the cambium layer hurts the tree and can kill it.

The most delicious gifts of the conifers, especially the pines, are the seeds. Pinecones ripen in fall and produce tons of fatty, nutritious seeds that can be eaten raw or roasted. The piñon pines of the West release large, easily harvested and nuts in commercial quantities. When the nuts are ripe, the cones simply open and spill them out. (You can pry out the seeds when unripe as well, but they're not as tasty.) Other species have smaller fruits that require more energy to harvest. Some have closed scales that must be cut or pried open or heated in a fire to reveal the nuts inside.

The central core of unripe, green pinecones may also be roasted and eaten. The pine pitch has been chewed as gum (and heated for glue).

Grasses

Just about all grasses are edible at certain stages of growth, but with the exception of a few such as bamboo, they are so small that they aren't worth your while except in times of true starvation. The very young, tender shoots of springtime can be eaten before they have developed their stringy cellulose fibers, or they may be chewed and the fibers spat out. The seeds are very nutritious, of course, and their cultivation has led to the development of civilization: wheat, corn, and rice are grasses. However, in the wild, grasses do not grow in orderly homogenous batches that ripen at almost exactly the same time and can be harvested all at once. Also, once they're gathered they must be threshed and winnowed (the outer husks removed and separated) before they can be used. Grasses are a practical food source for a village but much less so for a lone wilderness traveler.

Nettles

Stinging nettles are nutritious green vegetables that won't bite back once they're cooked. They grow by shady streamsides, sometimes reaching heights of 6 feet.

The stems are ribbed, the leaves are opposite on the stem and have serrated edges, and the whole plant is covered with soft hairs which are, in fact, hollow little needles filled with an irritating fluid that will raise burning, itching blisters on your skin if you brush against them. Once the young leaves and plant tops are tossed into boiling or steaming water, though, they immediately become harmless and delicious. Pick them with gloves and cook them like spinach. Native Americans used the stringy parts of the dried stems to make fine, but very strong, cordage.

Docks

There are several different plants known as dock in the genus *Rumex*. Some are wonderfully tangy, like salad with a bit of lemon juice built in; some are downright bitter; others are somewhere in between. Their tang comes from oxalic acid, which is harmless in moderate quantities. The most popular are sheep sorrel and curly dock.

Sheep sorrel rarely grows taller than 18 inches, is usually found in dry, disturbed soil, and is easily recognized by its arrowhead-shaped leaves. Eat it raw or cooked.

Curly dock is also found in dry places along roadsides and abandoned fields. It gets much taller than sheep sorrel, up to 4 feet. Its leaves are long and slender, especially toward the base of the plant, and its edges are wavy rather than curly. It may be eaten like sheep sorrel.

The stems of both kinds of dock sometimes have a reddish tinge. Both plants produce long, narrow stalks above the leaves where hundreds of tiny, inconspicuous flowers are clustered. The flowers are green when young, then turn reddish brown when the seeds develop. These are easy to strip from the plant and make wonderful nutty-flavored flour when threshed and winnowed, but they are not useful for short-term survival. (The docks are very effective antidotes to nettle stings, too. Crush the leaves and rub them on your skin before the blisters have a chance to develop.)

EDIBLE INSECTS

Insects are more nutritious than plants, are extremely plentiful, and are eaten with relish by people all over the world. Their only disadvantage as a survival food is their small size. If you can gather enough of them without expending too much energy, go for it. Scrape off the top couple of inches from a patch of damp, loosely packed soil for earthworms. Rotting logs are often seething with fat, delicious larvae, but you need a hatchet or similar tool to get to them. It's a good idea to cook any insects you catch before eating them. Many harbor parasites that might make you sick, though bug meat in itself is usually safe.

CONCLUSION

Practice Survival and You Will Survive

The key to survival is the confidence that comes from preparation and practice. Practice your survival skills before an emergency arises so you won't be taken by surprise or give in to destructive panic. Once you're aware of the kinds of situations that might confront you in the wilderness and are comfortable with your ability to deal with them, you're bound to have a more enjoyable outdoor experience every time.

As a bonus, you'll find that your sense of confidence will communicate itself to your companions and make everybody less subject to panic when that rare emergency arises. In addition, you'll have the satisfaction of knowing you won't add to the current strain on the resources of public agencies and rescue organizations.

About the Author

Suzanne Swedo has conducted wilderness survival, outdoor skills, and natural science outings for over twenty-five years as founder and director of WILD, an international and domestic adventure travel company. She has also led trips for nonprofit educational organizations, including Wilderness Institute, Pacific Wilderness Institute, Outdoor Adventures, Sierra Club, and University of California Extension. She teaches backcountry natural history seminars for the Yosemite Association in Yosemite National Park, and served as survival consultant to the ten-week Warner Brothers television series *Alive and Well.* Her writings on survival have appeared in such publications as the *Los Angeles Examiner* and *California* magazine. She is the author of the FalconGuides *Adventure Travel Tips, Best Easy Day Hikes Yosemite, Hiking California's Golden Trout Wilderness,* and *Hiking Yosemite National Park.*